Chinese dietary wisdom
Eating for health and wellbeing

GW00671733

The digestive system and Spleen in Chinese medicine

Claire never eats breakfast. She's trying to lose weight. She feels tired and jumpy at work so she grabs a latte mid-morning and then has a quick half-sandwich whilst shopping at lunchtime. By 3 o'clock she's exhausted and that box of biscuits is too hard to resist. After a year of living like this, Claire has put on a stone, struggles to get to sleep and is battling with depression. Ten years later the doctor prescribes medication for diabetes and that's when Claire decides her body has turned against her.

It's surprising how little we stop to think about our eating habits as life races along. This book is designed to share some of Chinese medicine's ancient knowledge about how to look after our digestive system for optimal health.

Westerners are often surprised to hear that Chinese medicine places our Spleen* at the centre of the digestive process. After all, doctors tell us that we can survive perfectly well without a spleen at all. The 'Spleen' of Chinese medicine theory is the name given to the set of energetic functions that make up our entire digestive process.

The Spleen is the digestive fire of the body. Its job is to transform our food into energy (Qi) and transport it around our body to nourish us physically, mentally and emotionally.

If the Spleen is strong then digestion will be strong, metabolism will be effective and we will be able to adapt to our food and our environment. If the Spleen is weak, metabolism may become slow and sluggish; we may become overweight, or start to experience digestive problems such as loose bowels and bloating.

But here's the good news: tending to the Spleen is largely down to us. There are simple rules to keep the digestive fire burning consistently. Enough warmth and movement is essential for this process. Looking after the Spleen will prevent the digestive process from becoming Stagnant, potentially leading to heaviness, bloating and muddled thinking.

* When we refer to an organ using a capital letter (Spleen, Liver, Heart, Lung, Kidney), we are talking about a broad range of energetic functions from a Chinese medicine perspective, not just the biomedical organ itself. We have also given initial caps to other Chinese medicine terms to distinguish them from biomedical and other meanings.

General principles
of healthy eating
from a Chinese medicine perspective

In traditional Chinese medicine it is not only what we eat that is important, but also when and how we eat. The best diet for you is also dependent on many factors (lifestyle, constitution, metabolism, strength of digestive system), and differs widely from person to person. This section gives a general guide to healthy eating.

Your Chinese medicine practitioner may highlight the advice in this section which is most relevant to you.

Before considering any of the suggestions, remember that food is a blessing. Enjoying food and having a good relationship with food is of the utmost importance. Try to remain mindful of when, how and what you eat. The best food is homegrown, home cooked with love, and enjoyed around a table in good company.

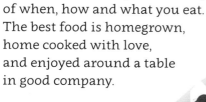

When we eat

'Breakfast like a king, lunch like a prince and dine like a pauper'
Our digestive systems are at their strongest between 7 and 9am and their weakest between 7 and 9pm. Eat a good, hearty breakfast (for example porridge, muesli or a cooked breakfast). This really is the most important meal of the day.

Avoid eating late at night Your digestive system can't cope with a large meal when your metabolism is already slowing down. In the short term this will overburden your digestive system, possibly disturbing your sleep. The food will sit, undigested, in your system and can make you feel disinterested in food, sluggish, groggy, and slightly nauseous in the morning. In the long term it may deplete the digestive fluids and weaken the digestive system.

If you are eating, just eat Your blood can only be in one place at a time. Whilst eating, it is needed in your digestive system. If you are doing something else, your blood will be diverted to another part of your body, and you will be less able to digest. If you stand or walk, blood will be diverted to your legs. If you watch television, read, drive or work, blood will be diverted to your brain. For this reason eating on the go, business lunches and TV dinners are all best avoided.

Stay relaxed while you are eating Eating while stressed, nervous or uptight may lead to food Stagnating in your digestive system. In the long term this may lead to digestive problems like heartburn or ulcers. Mealtimes are definitely not the time for family arguments!

The stomach likes regularity Try to make your mealtimes as regular as possible, as your body will prepare for digestion. Avoid missing meals (which may weaken the digestive fluids), constant snacking (which could lead to Stagnation in the digestive system) and eating late. Diabetics are only too aware of the need to eat a regular sensible diet to maintain healthy blood sugar levels.

Take time to digest Your body needs time to digest once you have eaten your food. Try not to rush on to the next thing but instead take a little while to digest your food and relax. Avoid indigestion.

How we eat

Don't drown your food Healthy digestion requires an abundance of digestive fluids. Drinking a large quantity of fluid with your meals will water down these powerful digestive juices. Instead have a small amount of fluid with a meal and drink the rest of your fluids between meals.

Don't chill your stomach Your digestive system needs a level of 'Heat' to digest food in just the same way that we need to cook food. For this reason avoid food directly from the fridge and try not to have iced drinks with your food. Avoid over-eating raw food if your digestive system is already weak. Instead lightly steam or stir-fry vegetables to make them more digestible without losing valuable nutrients. Cooking soups and stews is a good way to retain more of the goodness from vegetables.

The stomach has no teeth Digestion starts in the mouth. Make sure that you chew your food well, even soup. Eat slowly so that your system has time to digest.

Avoid overeating Stop before you get totally full. Eating slowly helps prevent overeating – the stomach takes a while to give the brain the message that it is full. You wouldn't expect your washing machine to wash if you crammed it totally full of clothes – how can you expect your digestive system to do the same?

Listen to your own body We know intuitively what food is good for us, and which foods keep us healthy. The multitude of advice in the form of diets, science, news (and books like this) can undermine our own ability to know what is good for us. How does your body feel (before, during and after) eating different foods? Remain mindful, listen carefully, and learn to trust your body.

Cravings Craving for sweet foods and carbs may be a sign that your digestive system is weak – it wants easy energy without having to work hard to digest the food. Make sure that you are getting plenty of foods that will maintain a steady blood sugar level (like oats or brown rice). Craving for salty food may mean that you are low in some minerals. We sometimes crave the very foods that are doing us harm, and we may need to eliminate this food entirely for a while.

Larger issues Try to make yourself aware of the larger issues involved in the farming of food and make well-informed choices. Find out more about locally produced, fairtrade, ethically produced, and organic food. Take responsibility for how the food you eat is produced and transported.

What we eat

Choose food with strong Qi (vital energy) Always choose fresh above processed food. Choose good quality or organic over non-organic and poor quality. Choose locally-grown in-season food whenever possible. Avoid over-processed and pre-packaged food. The extra money and time that this takes is well worth it.

Eat appropriate proportions Our diet should consist mostly of vegetables and good quality carbohydrates (like wholegrain rice, pasta, potatoes with skins and oats), with a smaller part (roughly 20–30%) of high protein foods (such as meat, dairy and eggs) and fats. It is important to include fruit (one to three pieces per day). Imagine this on a plate; the largest portion should be vegetables, followed by carbs, with the smallest segment being protein food. This of course varies depending on age and levels of activity. Imagine these proportions in the following foods: a pizza; soup and bread; pesto pasta; a roast dinner; a burger and salad. Which of these meals contain the appropriate proportions? How could you modify them to redress the balance – a side salad or side plate of vegetables, perhaps?

Eat a balanced diet/avoid extremes Foods that are relatively bland and neutral should make up the bulk of our diet, while foods that are more extreme in nature (strongly flavoured, rich, greasy, spicy, salty or sweet) should make up a small part of what we eat. This means that very concentrated and refined foods (like sugar and fruit juice) should only be consumed occasionally.

Avoid over-consuming any one food It is not unusual for somebody to eat a wheat-based breakfast cereal, a sandwich for lunch, and pasta for their evening meal – resulting in most of the diet consisting of wheat. This is not a balanced diet!

Variety is the spice of life Eat a wide range of different foods rather than sticking to the same old things. Try to eat a range of different coloured vegetables (red, orange, green, purple, yellow) with every meal. Not only does this look appealing, but you will be getting a good range of nutrients. Many of the colour pigments in food (yellows and oranges: beta-carotene; greens and whites: indoles; reds and pinks: lycopenes; blues and deep reds: anthocyanins) are thought to have a strong effect in boosting the immune system.

Avoid unnecessary additives Try to minimise as much as possible food additives such as sweeteners, preservatives, colourings and flavourings. Homemade food is usually better and you can tailor it to suit your needs.

Choose good quality oils Rapeseed oil, butter, ghee and coconut oil are great for cooking (as are hard animal fats in small amounts); extra virgin olive oil and flax seed oil are great for salad dressings; avoid overeating the poor quality hydrogenated vegetable fats and margarine often found in processed foods and foods with long shelf lives. If bacteria don't want to eat it, you probably don't either!

Choose the best meat you can afford Reduce preserved or smoked meats (such as salami, bacon and ham) and choose local or organic meat. If price is an issue, eat less meat but go for good quality.

Drink plenty of water We are designed to drink water, and water should be available as often as possible – a bottle in your backpack, a glass on your desk. Fizzy drinks and fruit juices are usually full of sugar, and should only be an occasional treat. Tea, coffee and hot chocolate should not be over-consumed – replace them with hot water, herbal teas, or milder green and white teas.

Use lots of digestives Use plenty of digestives in your cooking to aid gut motility and improve your digestive process. This includes natural probiotics (such as yoghurt, sauerkraut or miso), herbs (including most aromatic herbs, pepper, coriander, basil and cumin) and pickles.

Eating with the seasons

Eat appropriately to the season Our diet should be modified to suit the time of year – the simplest way to do this is to eat food that is in season.

More nourishment in the autumn/winter In the winter, our system needs a richer diet, with more protein, to keep our bodies warm and energised. To help us digest these richer foods, we also need more digestives, such as herbs and gentle spices. Warming cooking methods such as casseroles, stews, roasting and soups should be chosen, and salads and cold foods should be reduced.

Lighter food in the spring/summer In the summer our diet should be lighter and cooler. Leaves, flowers, and watery vegetables are more abundant and should be eaten more. Choose cooling cooking methods such as stir-frying, steaming and grilling and reduce deep-fried and roasted food. Some raw food (salads) with suitable dressings can be added, and fruit can be increased.

Maintaining and losing weight

Follow the general principles Eat appropriate proportions at suitable times as described above, and you will reach and maintain an appropriate weight for your body type. It is especially important to maintain a good relationship with food and to practise 'mindful eating' – do not make food the enemy.

Consider the calories A calorie is a scientific measure of how much Qi or energy is contained in a food. Rich and fatty foods tend to have more calories, with vegetables containing the lowest. By eating healthily and maintaining appropriate proportions of food, calories are automatically controlled. Be aware of portion sizes, chew food well, eat slowly, and stop eating before feeling completely full. Avoid high calorie drinks (including alcohol and juice) and refined carbohydrates and sugar. Increase the amount of vegetables you eat to keep you feeling full without increasing calories. Replacing your regular plate and bowl with smaller ones will help keep portion sizes down.

Exercise and weight loss It is very hard to 'exercise' weight off without changing diet – a 40-minute walk or a 20-minute run or swim will only use roughly the amount of calories in a packet of crisps. However, exercise improves metabolism (increases Yang), increases muscle mass and will help you to lose weight in the long term. As well as regular exercise, try to incorporate fitness into your daily life – walk up the stairs, cycle to work, go for a stroll, bake some handmade bread!

A traditional approach In Chinese medicine, weight gain is considered to be Phlegm and Dampness, often caused not only by diet, but also by a weak digestive system (Spleen Qi Deficiency) or slow metabolism (Kidney Yang Deficiency), and successful nutritional advice might be aimed at these conditions. Eat three meals a day at regular times. Missing meals will further deplete your digestive system and predispose you to more weight gain. Try to avoid snacking, especially in the evening.

Getting more fruit and veg into your daily diet

Aim to eat 40% or more

Beautiful presentation Try this experiment. First, put a fruit bowl out after dinner – how much gets eaten? Next try chopping up a few pieces of fruit into bite sized pieces, and arrange it on a plate beautifully before putting it out – how much gets eaten now?

Hide healthy veg in sauces Make a tomato sauce – fry onions and garlic, add tomatoes, stock and herbs and simmer it down. You can add virtually any veg to this – try mushrooms, pepper, spinach or courgette. Fry it up with the onions; add enough tomato purée to bring the colour back to a nice red, and season well with suitable herbs and spices. This versatile sauce can form the basis of a pizza topping, a pasta sauce, a chilli, a filling for jacket potatoes, and so on.

Serve healthy sides Serve every meal with a side dish of veg, salad, or have vegetable soup as a starter. If time is short buy a mixture of frozen veg to reboil. Experiment with cooked salads adding griddled, steamed or roasted veg such as squash, fennel or courgette to your salads. If you are eating out regularly, order a children's sized portion with an extra portion of vegetables.

Find healthier alternatives Replace sandwiches with soups and cooked salads; buy a food flask, and take your left-overs to work for lunch; make healthy snacks such as chopped vegetables with a dip, seed mixes or vegetable sushi.

Try adding one more portion Add berries and chopped fruit to your muesli, yoghurt or porridge. Change your snack to fresh or dried fruit. Replace potatoes with other root vegetables like beetroots, swede, carrots and parsnips. Blend cooked pepper or carrot into your hummus.

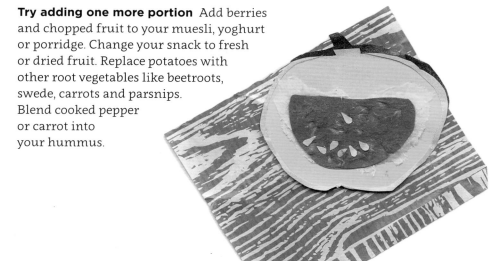

Food types with recipes

The following food types are described from a Chinese medicine viewpoint. Chinese medicine describes food energetically. It does this through the eight flavours (sweet, salty, sour, pungent, bitter, aromatic, bland and spicy); the five temperatures (cool, cold, neutral, warm and hot); and the Organ resonances (for example, the Spleen).

We've included some recipe ideas to inspire you. Temperatures are for fan-assisted ovens (increase by 20°C for conventional ovens, or convert for gas). Use a measuring cup that holds approximately 250ml of liquid.

Fruit

From a Chinese medicine perspective fruit tends to cool the body, making it perfect summer food – two or three portions per day are a great addition to our diet. Fruit's sweet and sour flavour nourishes the Yin – the fluids of the body, and hence has a moistening and laxative effect. It can clear Heat and Toxins from the body – people with a hangover often crave fruit. Because of its cooling and laxative nature, too much can overcool the digestive system, and some fruit (bananas, oranges, fruit juice) can aggravate Damp and Phlegm. Cooking or drying fruit makes it warmer and easier to digest (especially with some digestive herbs like ginger and cinnamon). Juicing fruit makes it cooler, sweeter, and harder on the digestive system, and should only be used as an occasional treat. Overeating fruit (especially as fruit juice) can overload our systems with sugar (fruit sugar has to be broken down by the liver) so as always moderation is the key to a healthy diet.

Tropical fruits and very acidic fruits (pineapples, gooseberries) are Colder and harder to digest than our native fruits (apples, pears). Berries (raspberry, blackberry, blueberry, bilberry, cranberry, wolfberry) are full of bioflavonoids, which may enhance our immune system, and are a great addition to our diets.

Smoothies and juices Try to blend rather than juice whenever possible to conserve valuable fibre and nutrition, and include vegetables such as beetroot, kale, carrot and celery. Digestive herbs (such as fresh ginger and parsley) make great additions to a juice. Never add ice, and serve at room temperature to aid digestion. Yoghurt, seeds, nuts and oats can all be added to make a more balanced drink. Drink your smoothies through a straw to save your teeth.

Breakfast smoothie

Smoothies are perfect if you just can't tolerate food in the morning and need to retrain your body to want breakfast. If you need to gain weight, add cow's milk and nuts to the mix and use as a snack between meals.
1 Mix together one chopped banana, one cup of rice milk (cow's, coconut, soya or almond milk also work well), ¼ to ½ cup of fresh or frozen berries (use less blueberries, and more strawberries or raspberries), ¼ cup porridge oats, ½ tsp vanilla essence. **2** Blend all the ingredients together. Add nuts or seeds (cashews or sunflower seeds work well) for a bit of crunch.

Baked pears

1 Halve and core 4–5 firm pears and lay face down in a pan. **2** Make a syrup by boiling 3 tbsp honey, ¼ tsp cinnamon, 2 tbsp sugar and ½ tsp vanilla essence with a cup of water. **3** Pour over the pears and bake in a 180°C oven for 20–30 minutes until soft. **4** Serve with crème fraiche or yoghurt.

Nuts and seeds

Nuts and seeds have a dense, heavy nature – lots of potential in a tiny package – and strengthen our energy (Qi) and in some cases our reserves (Jing). Their natural sweetness nourishes the Qi, and their heavy oily nature moistens the bowels (lots of fibre) and has a grounding/settling effect. Their high levels of minerals (such as zinc, magnesium, copper and vitamin E) and other goodies (the 'good' fats) perhaps explain why they make such great tonics for the Qi, Blood, Yin and Yang. Peanuts are not nuts at all, and their rich oily nature can easily aggravate Damp and Phlegm – as can too many nuts generally, especially old nuts that are starting to go rancid.

Toasted seeds

These seeds are delicious on their own as a snack, and make a great topping for a salad. **1** Get a good handful of pumpkin seeds and sunflower seeds, and dry roast them in a heavy frying pan. **2** When they start to brown and pop, give them a light covering of soy sauce, stir in, and remove from the heat.

Crispbread

This tasty snack is dairy, sugar and wheat free. **1** Mix together 1 cup of maize/corn flour, ½ cup of sunflower seeds, ¼ cup each of sesame seeds, pumpkin seeds and golden linseeds, ¼ cup olive or rapeseed oil, 1¼ cups warm water and 1 tsp salt. **2** Mix the goo together and spread a thin layer over two greased baking trays. **3** Cook in a 150°C oven for an hour – your crispbreads will be beautifully golden, crisp and ready to eat hot or cold.

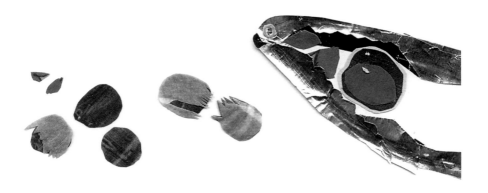

Almond moments

Almonds are a useful tonic for our energy (Qi) and reserves (Jing), whilst being less Phlegm and Damp forming than many other nuts.
1 Put 1 cup almonds, ½ cup sunflower seeds and 1 cup mixed dried fruit (cranberries, apricots, dates, raisins) in a blender, and blend into small pieces. **2** Add enough honey to bind the mix. **3** Squeeze into small balls (put a sandwich bag over your hand to stop them sticking). You can roll them in desiccated coconut if you like to keep them drier.

Pine nut and walnut pesto

Both nuts nourish and moisten the Lung and Large Intestine. Use in moderation when Phlegm is present. **1** Lightly roast a small handful each of pine nuts and walnuts. **2** Blend these in a processor with a handful of Parmesan cheese, a large chopped clove of garlic, two good handfuls of fresh basil and a slurp of your best olive oil. Whilst mixing, add more olive oil to create your desired consistency and season with salt and pepper. **3** Stir into pasta, couscous, quinoa, rice or other grains.

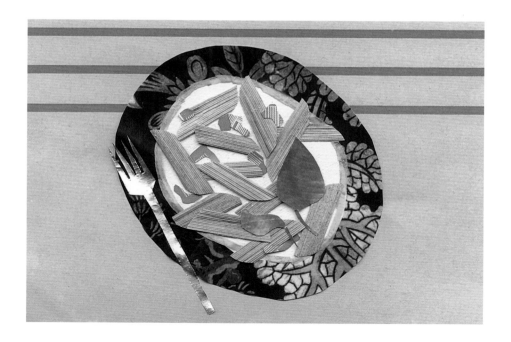

Grains

Grains are the seeds of grasses, and can be highly nutritious, nourishing Qi and Blood and ensuring a slow, steady release of energy. Always choose wholegrain varieties wherever possible. It is said in the classical texts of Chinese medicine that 'grains build and vegetables cleanse'. Their gentle sweet nature strengthens our Qi, their high fibre content helps to drain Dampness and keep the intestines clean. They have a calming, grounding nature said to promote clear thinking. They require lots of chewing for proper digestion, especially whole grains. Avoid overeating grains, especially wheat and bread, and avoid cheap refined grains as much as possible. Try varying wheat with other grains such as oats or rye – or use quinoa or amaranth (not strictly speaking true grains) as a highly nutritious alternative.

Quinoa tabouleh

1 Dry roast 1 cup of quinoa in a heavy saucepan for 30 seconds, then add 2 cups stock and boil for 20 minutes until tender. **2** Meanwhile, finely dice a mixture of vegetables – try cucumber, pepper, red onion and tomato, roughly the same amount as the cooked quinoa. **3** While the quinoa is still warm, mix in the veg (the heat of the quinoa will cook it just a little). **4** In a separate bowl mix the juice and zest of a lemon, ½ tsp salt, 2 tbsp flax or olive oil, 2 tsp cumin, a good handful of fresh chopped parsley or coriander, and a smaller handful of fresh mint. **5** Mix this with the cooled quinoa, and serve at room temperature.

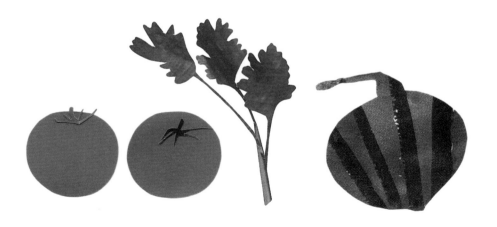

Breakfast granola

The sweet/bitter flavour of oats strengthens our energy (Qi) and has a calming, settling effect. They are thought to help to maintain healthy cholesterol levels. **1** Mix 1kg porridge oats (10 cups), 1 cup rapeseed or olive oil, ½ cup runny honey and 1 tsp vanilla essence, plus any nuts or seeds you like in a large bowl, and bake on two large oven trays in a 160°C oven for 15–20 minutes until lightly toasted, mixing half way through. **2** Mix together 3 cups of dried fruit – raisins, cranberries, blueberries, apricots, dates, or your own favourites. **3** Once cooled, combine the two mixtures evenly and store in an airtight container. **4** Serve with fresh fruit and cow's, rice or almond milk.

Oatcakes

Perfect served with your choice of spreads, hummus (page 17) or smoked mackerel and horseradish paté (page 22). **1** Mix 200g finely rolled oats with 50ml olive or coconut oil and 1 tsp good quality salt in a large bowl. **2** Pour on 2–3 tbsp boiling water to make a malleable dough. **3** On a floured surface roll out to about 5mm thick and cut to the shape you want – using a cutter helps. **4** Put the oatcakes on a lined baking tray and bake in a 160°C oven for around 15 minutes until they are a little browned. **5** Take out and allow to cool before eating.

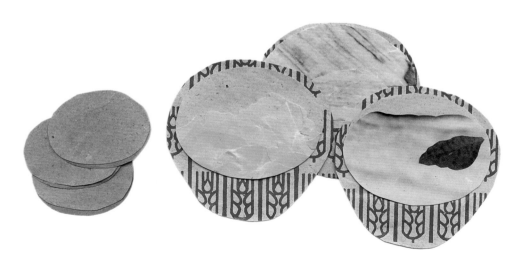

Beans and pulses (legumes)

Beans tend to be sweet and nourishing, but also drain Dampness and excess fluids from the body. Because of this they combine well with nourishing but moistening grains (making the 'complete protein' of a vegan diet). Dried pulses are notoriously difficult to digest: they need to be well washed and soaked, and cooked with lots of digestives such as ginger, cardamom or cumin to aid digestion (hence the garlic in hummus and the spices in dhal).

Aduki beans, mung beans, lentils and peas are the easiest to digest, and the best for regular consumption. Soya beans have been described as 'the beef of China' for their wonderful nourishing ability, but are best consumed in the easily digestible forms of tofu and miso. In Chinese herbal medicine, mung beans and tofu are thought to remove Toxins from the body.

Bean sprouts are more cooling than beans. Representing the most 'vital' stage of a plant's growth, they help to move Stagnant Qi, Detoxify and clear Heat from the system.

Pea and mint soup

Peas strengthen the digestive system, and provide lots of fibre, whilst both peas and mint help to move Stagnant Qi in the Liver and digestive system. **1** Brown a diced onion in a little butter. **2** Add 3 cups of peas (frozen or fresh), 3 cups of stock and ¼ cup fresh mint into a pan and boil until the peas are soft and well cooked. **3** Blend well, season with salt and pepper, and serve topped with yoghurt.

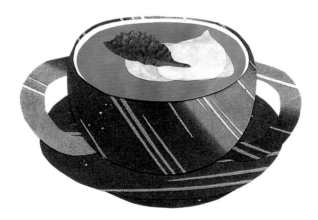

Easy dhal

Lentils are nourishing to the Qi (energy) and Jing (reserves) and this dhal makes a simple and nourishing lunch. It is well seasoned to give both a great flavour, and to aid digestion of the lentils. **1** Soak and wash 1½ cups of lentils and get them simmering gently, removing any residue that forms on the top. **2** Brown a diced onion in some oil, then mix in 1 tsp each of cumin and coriander powder and ¼ tsp turmeric, adding this to the lentils after a minute or two. **3** Cook for 20–30 minutes until the lentils are soft. Add enough water as the lentils cook to prevent sticking. Blend the mix if you prefer a smooth dhal. **4** Fry 2 thinly cut slices of garlic and 1 tsp cumin seeds until they start to brown, and add this to your dhal before seasoning. **5** Serve with rice and pickle.

Easy hummus

Chickpeas and black soybeans both nourish the vital Qi of Spleen and Kidney. For black soybean hummus, replace the chickpeas with a can of black soybeans and the lemon juice with a similar quantity of soy sauce.
1 Place the chickpeas from a 400g tin in a food processor, keeping the fluid for later. **2** Add 1 finely chopped clove of garlic, 1 tbsp of tahini, juice of ½ a good-sized lemon and 1 tbsp olive oil, and blend. **3** Add some of the fluid from the can as you mix, to make a consistency that is smooth and a little runny. **4** Season with salt, black pepper, cayenne or paprika to your taste.

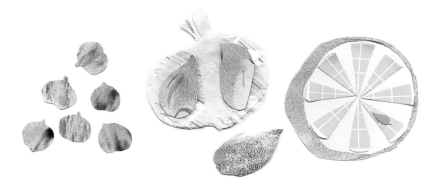

Vegetables

It is said that 'grains build, vegetables cleanse' and together they should make up the bulk of our diet. Raw veg is the most cleansing, but is hard work for the digestion, and is most suitable during hotter weather, in moderate amounts. Cooked vegetables are more nourishing and easier to digest. Vegetable juice is Colder still, and is best as an occasional addition for most people. If you do juice, choose a juicer that blends the pulp rather than discarding it.

Root vegetables tend to be sweet and nourish Qi and Blood – the edible part is the plant's own store of Qi (energy) to get it through the winter. Roots are the easiest foods to digest, and are especially good for infants and the very weak.

Carrots, celeriac, parsnips, celery and fennel are all great digestive tonics. Carrots aid vision (they contain beta-carotene, converted by the body to vitamin A – an important nutrient for eye health). Celery clears Liver Heat and helps maintain a good blood pressure. [1]

Potatoes have a grounding nourishing nature craved by many. Along with the other solanaceae (peppers, aubergine and tomatoes) they contain low doses of solanine, which some people find aggravates rheumatic conditions. Sweet potatoes, squash and pumpkin are more nourishing, and make a great alternative to starchy potatoes.

Dark green leafy vegetables tend to nourish Blood and move a Stagnant Liver. Alliums' pungent nature (onions, garlic, chives, spring onions and leeks) helps to move Stagnant Qi, activate the Lungs, and they are useful as digestives. Garlic is useful for controlling parasites (including candida). Some religions consider alliums too Heating and 'stimulating to the desires' to consume, and use asafoetida instead as a digestive and flavouring.

Watery vegetables (like courgettes and cucumbers) tend to be cooling and moistening (they nourish Yin fluids).

Fast growing foods and tips (like asparagus and spinach) tend to be Colder than slower growing vegetables.

Brassicas (such as cabbages, cauliflower, sprouts, turnips and kohlrabi) have a sweet but slightly peppery flavour, and a neutral nature, which helps to both nourish and move our digestive systems, making them ideal vegetables for regular consumption. They also mildly nourish the Blood. Modern research indicates that they may be useful for inhibiting intestinal cancers. [2]

Mushrooms help to clear Phlegm and Damp from the system, clear Toxins, and boost the immune system (especially shiitake mushrooms). [3, 4]

Vegetable soup

Soup is a great way to get lots of nutritious, well-cooked and easily digested vegetables into your diet. It is perfect for lunch, freezes well (freeze it in portion-sized pots) and has long been used for people who are weak or convalescing. Season it well, and make your own stock if you have time. Here is a basic method. Follow steps 1–5 to make any of our favourite soups listed below, or experiment with your own variations

Basic vegetable soup recipe

The onions, garlic and herbs/spices act as digestives, add flavour, and change the energetics of the soup. **1** Fry onions and garlic in a little oil until translucent. **2** Add herbs and spices, and allow them to fry until aromatic (1–2 minutes). **3** Add vegetables peeled, prepared, chopped and diced. **4** Add liquid, bring to the boil and simmer (lid on) until cooked. **5** Blend if necessary, season with salt, pepper. Serve with a topping as described in the recipes below.

Spiced parsnip soup

Parsnips nourish our digestive energy (Spleen Qi), while the milk nourishes our Yin. The Heating herbs and spices aid the parsnips to make this a Yang warming soup and aid the digestion of the milk. **1** 1 onion, 2 cloves garlic. **2** ½ fresh chilli, 25 mm peeled and diced fresh ginger, 1 tsp each coriander, cumin, garam masala. **3** 5–6 parsnips. **4** 2 cups stock, 1½ cups milk; simmer for 20–25 minutes. **5** Blend thoroughly and season.

Smooth fennel soup

Fennel's sweet and slightly spicy flavour strengthens the Qi and the digestive system, whilst its warm nature warms and moves stuck energy (Qi). **1** 1 onion. **2** ½ tsp fennel seeds. **3** 1 fennel head, 3 carrots. **4** 3 cups stock; simmer for 20 minutes. **5** Blend thoroughly and season well.

Carrot and coriander soup

Carrots strengthen the digestive energy (Qi) and help keep the body free of parasites. Coriander moves Qi and along with the lime zest, acts as a digestive. This classic soup is nourishing and full of flavour.
1 1 onion, 2 cloves garlic. **3** 6 carrots, 2 potatoes. **4** 2–3 cups stock; simmer for 20 minutes. **5** Add a good handful of fresh coriander (15g), and the zest of 1 lime. Blend until smooth. Serve topped with fresh yoghurt.

Beetroot and wasabi soup

Beetroot nourishes and harmonises the Blood, the carrots support this role and strengthen the Qi. The wasabi activates the digestive system.
1 1 onion, 1 clove garlic. **2** ¼ tsp wasabi or 1 tsp horseradish.
3 3 medium beetroot, 3 carrots. **4** 3 cups stock; simmer for 20-30 minutes.
5 Blend smooth and season well. Serve topped with fresh yoghurt.

Chunky tomato and pesto soup

Tomatoes and celery nourish Yin and fluids, and help to clear Heat, while the herbs and spices aid the digestion, making for a light cooling summer soup. Celery particularly clears Liver Heat.
1 1 onion, 1 clove garlic. **2** 1 tsp oregano, 1 tsp paprika.
3 1 pepper, 3 tomatoes, 2 sticks of celery, 2 carrots, 1 leek or any mix of similar summer veg. **4** 2 cans of chopped tomatoes (400g cans, or 10 fresh), 2 cups stock, 1 tin butterbeans, washed (400g tin); simmer for 20-30 minutes. **5** Blend roughly or leave chunky. Dollop a spoon of homemade pesto on top – see recipe on page 13.

Spiced roast vegetables

The warm and pungent herbs in this help to move stuck Qi. Some herbs also activate blood circulation. **1** Choose your vegetables and chop to easy bite-sized pieces (peppers, aubergines, courgettes, butternut squash, fennel or leeks, cauliflower, onions). **2** Layer in a pan so not squashed.
3 Lightly coat with olive oil along with a choice of the following: whole cloves of garlic, bay, cayenne, cinnamon, fennel, turmeric or star anise.
4 Mix well with your hands adding some salt to your taste.
5 Roast at 180°C for 45 minutes, stirring well once after 20 minutes.
Eat warm or leave to cool and add to salads or have in your lunchbox.

Meat and animal products

Red meat is very rich and nourishing, and tends to be warm, sweet and often salty. It is the most Blood nourishing food, especially for very deficient constitutions, those recovering from an illness, or after a pregnancy. Its rich and fatty nature can easily cause Stagnation and Heat, so it is best eaten in small amounts. Animal organs and offal are very nourishing, and a useful addition to our diet (choosing good quality, reliably sourced and ideally organic is especially important here). Frying or roasting makes meat more Heating and harder to digest, whereas cooking meat in well-seasoned stews or casseroles aids the digestive process. Chicken is the mildest meat, and most suitable for regular consumption. Choose fresh and good quality meats over processed, smoked and preserved meats (such as bacon, sausages or salami).

Chicken soup for convalescing

The warming and nourishing effect of this Qi and Blood tonic makes it ideal for building up reserves. Traditionally used after an illness or childbirth, but useful anytime you need a good pick-me-up.
1 In a big pan lightly fry a large diced onion, two chopped cloves of garlic and a knob of finely chopped fresh ginger in a little olive oil.
2 Add 1kg of any mix of the following cut into bite-sized chunks: sweet potato, sweetcorn, carrots, peas, broad beans, broccoli and leeks.
3 Add 4 bay leaves and a small handful of flat parsley and thyme. Sauté over a medium heat for a few minutes. **4** Add 1 litre of the best chicken stock you can get (see below)and bring to the boil. **5** Simmer (lid on) for 45 minutes. **6** At this point you can either whizz the mix up to create a thicker soup or leave as is. **7** Add about 750g of chicken (a mixture of brown and white meat) and season with salt and pepper.

Chicken stock

There are some reasonable pre-made organic stocks available. Alternatively you can prepare this base stock in advance for later use. **1** Combine in a big pan 2.5kg chicken bones, gizzards (you can use the carcasses from your roasts), 200g each carrot, leek, celery, onion, 3 bay leaves, 6 dates, a sprig of thyme, 10 black peppercorns and 3 litres of water. **2** Bring to the boil and simmer (lid on) for 2–3 hours. Strain and leave to cool. **3** Skim off any fat and transfer to small containers for freezing.

Dairy products and eggs

Milk and cheese tend to be sweet, rich and very nourishing to the Yin (especially the Lungs). Because of this it can easily create Dampness and Phlegm, and is hard to digest. Goat's and sheep's milk and cheese tend to be warmer and easier to digest, and hence less Damp/Phlegm forming, than cow's. Spices like cardamom, ginger and nutmeg help to make milk more digestible. Butter is sweet and warming, helping Blood circulation, and clearing Cold from the system. Yoghurt and cottage cheese is fermented – this process makes it both easier to digest and a useful probiotic. Intolerance to milk may lead to abdominal cramps, wind, and loose bowels.[5] Eggs are sweet, neutral, and very nourishing to the Yin. The yolk can nourish our reserves (Jing). Overeating eggs can block us up and lead to Phlegm production.

Omelette

An excellent quick tonic to boost Yin and Jing reserves. Coriander leaves, marjoram or spring onions help balance the heaviness of the eggs. You can separate the eggs, whisk the whites until stiff, then blend in the yolks before you start to make it extra fluffy. **1** Whisk two or three fresh eggs. **2** Prepare your fillings – fresh herbs like coriander, parsley, tarragon and chives are excellent with the veg, cheese and/or meat of your choice. **3** Heat a 20 cm pan, add a nob of butter or olive oil then the whisked eggs and continue to whisk/scramble in the pan for a couple of seconds whilst keeping a cover of egg on the bottom of the pan. **4** Add your choice of fillings along with a pinch of salt and pepper **5** Flip in half while the egg consistency is still slightly runny. **6** Slide onto a plate alongside your choice of vegetables.

Seafood

The sweet, salty flavour of fish makes it deeply nourishing and Phlegm clearing, and its cooling nature makes a good counterbalance to eating lots of Heating rich meat. Shellfish tends to be more warming and Yang strengthening, and may lead to Heat reactions or aggravate skin conditions and inflammation in some people.

Smoked mackerel and horseradish paté

Mackerel is rich in quality oils and nourishes Yin. Try with baked potatoes and salad. **1** Place 2 good quality mackerel fillets (check for bones) in a food processor with 2 tsps horseradish sauce and 1 well-rounded tbsp of yoghurt or crème fraiche. **2** Blitz for a few seconds so the mix still has texture. **3** Add salt, pepper and the juice of ½ a lemon to taste.

Herbs and spices

Herbs and spices are strongly flavoured and hence are used in small amounts. They flavour and purify food, aid the digestive process, and are the simplest way to change the nature of a meal. Many of them can be used on their own medicinally (for example mint and ginger). Aromatic herbs 'awaken the digestive system'; pungent/spicy herbs move Qi and prevent Stagnation; bitter herbs dry Dampness; spicy/hot herbs warm the Yang. Some herbs can nourish in their own right – parsley is a useful Blood tonic as well as a digestive.

Aromatic and mildly spicy *Help to dry up Phlegm.* Basil, caraway, fennel seeds, fresh ginger, juniper, lemon zest, mustard, rosemary, tamarind, thyme. *Help to dry up Phlegm and transform Dampness.* Aniseed, cardamom, garlic, horseradish, pepper.

Hot/pungent *Warm up Cold constitutions, and activate the Yang; best eaten in moderate amounts.* Cayenne, chilli, cinnamon, raw garlic, dried ginger, horseradish, mustard, pepper.

Warm/pungent *Help to move stuck Qi (energy) and aid digestion. Some (bay, cayenne, chilli, nutmeg, turmeric, haws) also help Blood circulation.* Aniseed, basil, bay, caraway, cardamom, citrus peel, chive, clove, dill, fennel, fenugreek, juniper berries, marjoram, nutmeg, saffron, savory, star anise, thyme, turmeric.

Gently warming Yang tonics *Help to warm up Cold constitutions, aid digestion, and activate the Yang; suitable for regular consumption.* Basil, chive seed, clove, fennel seed, fenugreek, nutmeg, and rosemary.

Digestives *Help digest rich and difficult foods like meat, pulses or dairy.* Basil, cardamom, cinnamon, cloves, coriander, cumin, ginger, marjoram, mint, nutmeg, oregano, pepper, and thyme.

Herbal teas Chamomile helps to move the Qi, and is cooling and calming. Jasmine's sweet and slightly spicy flavour moves the Qi, lifts the spirit and clears Phlegm.

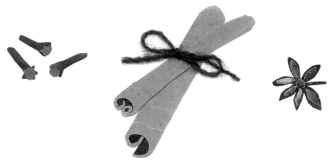

Making changes based on constitutional tendencies

The information in this section is only for use in the context of a full diagnosis and consultation with an acupuncturist or Chinese medicine practitioner. They will highlight the advice that is relevant to you, and you should ignore the rest.

The best changes are slow and gradual – change one thing a week.

The aim is always to return to a diet based around the general principles of healthy eating, see page 3 and food types, see page 10.

For ways to find a qualified practitioner near you, see page 48.

Wood patterns

Dietary advice

Lifestyle tips

LIVER BLOOD DEFICIENCY

Eat a relatively high proportion of protein foods (20–30% of your diet).

If you are vegetarian, ensure you eat 'complete proteins' (see Beans and pulses, page 16).

Chew food well and eat slowly in a relaxed environment.

Choose the best quality food that you can – locally produced and organic where possible, especially meat.

Preferred cooking methods are steaming, boiling, stewing and stir-frying.

Raw fruit and vegetables in small quantities.

Use a heavy iron frying pan.

Rest for a little after eating, especially after your main meal.

Take time to rest and recover after exercise.

For women...

It is important to rest more during and after your period, and if necessary to increase protein foods and iron rich foods at this time.

It can be helpful to lie down for 10 minutes at some point during the day and this especially applies if you have your period.

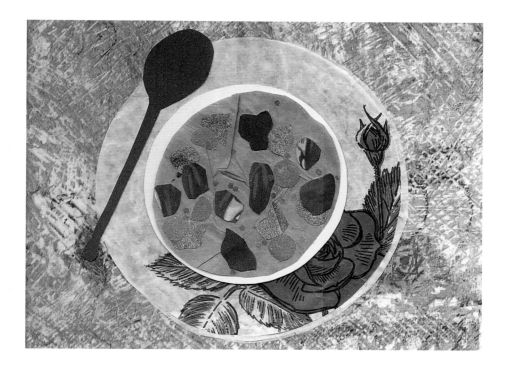

Beneficial foods

Leafy greens Cabbage and other brassicas, dandelion leaf, kale, kohlrabi, parsley, spinach, spring greens, watercress.

Animal products Chicken, chicken liver*, chicken eggs, quail and quail eggs, pork, pork liver*, lamb, lamb's liver*, beef, ox liver*, bone marrow, oysters, mussels, sardines, salmon.

Pulses and bean products Especially tofu, miso, mung beans, tempeh, aduki beans, black beans, kidney beans, haricot beans.

Fruit Apricots, cherries, dates, figs, goji berries, grapes, longan, lychee, mulberries, raisins.

Vegetables Alfalfa, avocado, beetroot, carrots, Chinese angelica, globe artichoke, tomatoes.

Grains Barley, brown rice, corn, oats.

Marmite, molasses, seaweed, sesame seeds, tahini, spirulina, wheatgerm.

* Except during pregnancy, due to high vitamin A

Foods to avoid or reduce

Fatty and deep-fried foods.

Processed foods.

Excessively salty or sweet foods.

Wood patterns continued

Dietary advice	Lifestyle tips

LIVER QI STAGNATION

Avoid overeating – stop before you feel completely full.

Chew food well and eat slowly.

Eat in a calm environment whenever possible.

Eat your main meal earlier in day.

Eat relatively fewer carbohydrates and proteins and more vegetables and fruit (40–50% of your diet).

Eat regularly, avoid missing meals and avoid snacking.

Use lots of herbs and aromatic spices in your cooking.

As far as possible restrict processed foods and choose fresh homemade food.

Regular exercise (of any type) is especially important. Go for a short walk soon after eating.

Get up, stretch and move around regularly, especially if you're sitting at work.

If you feel irritated, frustrated or tense, move!

LIVER FIRE

Eat plenty of raw foods, vegetable juices and salads.

Try to slow down, and remove yourself quickly from difficult situations or stressful environments.

Stay hydrated – water is best for this.

Also follow the advice given for Liver Qi Stagnation (above).

LIVER BLOOD STAGNATION

Follow the advice given for Liver Qi Stagnation (above).

A small amount of alcohol each day may be appropriate. Your Chinese medicine practitioner will advise on this.

Use lots of herbs and digestives in your cooking, especially turmeric.

Follow the advice given for Liver Qi Stagnation (above).

Beneficial foods	Foods to avoid or reduce

Mildly spicy (pungent) food Garlic, onions, radish, spring onion, mustard greens, watercress.

Herbs and spices Aniseed, basil, caraway, cardamom, coriander, cumin, citrus peel, chive, clove, dill, fennel, fenugreek, ginger, horseradish, juniper berries, marjoram, mint, nutmeg, pepper, saffron, savory, star anise, thyme, turmeric.

Sour foods Citrus (especially the zest), marmalade, pickles, vinegar in small amounts (especially cider vinegar).

Brassicas Cabbage, broccoli, cauliflower, sprouts, turnip, kale, kohlrabi.

Other fruit and veg Carrot, globe artichoke, mushroom, peach, peas, radish, squash.

Fatty and deep-fried foods
Dairy products (cheese, milk, cream), eggs, peanuts, chips, red meat, nuts, pastry.

Artificial preservatives, colouring, flavourings and additives.

Chocolate, recreational drugs, stimulants, excessive alcohol, coffee.

Processed foods.

Raw vegetables, vegetable juice and all fruits.

Sprouted grains, bean sprouts, mung beans, tofu.

All vegetables Especially celery, cucumber, lettuce, plums, rhubarb, spinach, tomatoes, water chestnut, watercress.

Herbal teas Peppermint, chamomile, mint or jasmine.

Fatty and deep-fried foods
Dairy products (cheese, milk, cream), eggs, peanuts, chips, red meat, nuts, pastry.

Artificial preservatives, colouring, flavourings and additives.

Chocolate, recreational drugs, stimulants, excessive alcohol, coffee.

Processed foods.

Alliums Chives, garlic, leek, onion, spring onion.

Herbs and spices Especially bay leaf, cayenne, chilli, coriander, hawthorn berry, mustard leaf, nutmeg, oregano, pepper, rosemary, turmeric.

Aduki bean, aubergine, buckwheat, caper, crab, green tea, kidney bean, peach, radish, red wine, seaweed, turnip, vinegar (in small amounts, especially cider vinegar).

Fatty and deep-fried foods
Dairy products (cheese, milk, cream), eggs, peanuts, chips, red meat, nuts, pastry.

Artificial preservatives, colouring, flavourings and additives.

Chocolate, recreational drugs, stimulants, excessive alcohol, coffee.

Processed foods.

Fire patterns

Dietary advice	Lifestyle tips

HEART BLOOD / YIN DEFICIENCY

Eat in a relaxed environment, and rest for a little after eating.

Eat slowly, and chew food well.

Preferred cooking methods are steaming, boiling, stewing and stir-frying.

Eat raw fruit and raw vegetables in small quantities only.

Consider meditation or relaxation to help overcome stressful and anxious states.

Useful activities include yoga, tai chi, qi gong, gardening or walking.

It is especially important to calm the body and mind in the evening before bed – create a routine that supports this when possible and prioritise switching off mobile devices and screens for at least an hour before you retire.

HEART QI / YANG DEFICIENCY

Avoid food and drinks directly from the fridge and anything cooler than room temperature.

Preferred cooking methods are steaming, stewing, boiling, baking and roasting.

Stay warm – keep well wrapped up.

Moderate exercise and regular movement is important. Exercising in a social environment can be especially helpful.

HEAT IN THE HEART / SHEN DISTURBED

Preferred cooking methods are raw food and salads, steaming, boiling and stewing.

Avoid overeating in the evening – it may be beneficial to eat your main meal earlier in the day.

Follow the advice given for Heart Blood/Yin Deficiency (above).

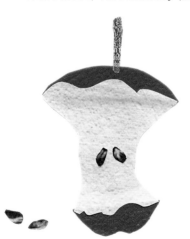

Beneficial foods	Foods to avoid or reduce

Leafy greens Cabbage and other brassicas, dandelion leaf, kale, kohlrabi, parsley, spinach, spring greens, watercress.

Vegetables Avocado, beetroot, carrots, Chinese angelica, globe artichoke.

Pulses and seeds Alfalfa, mung beans, aduki beans, sesame seeds and tahini.

Fruit Apricots, cherries, coconut and coconut products, dates, figs, goji berries, grapes, longan, lychee, mulberries, raisins.

Grains Wheatgerm, whole wheat, oats, brown rice, corn, barley.

Chicken, eggs, oyster, ginseng.

Coffee, alcohol, tobacco and other stimulants.

Hot and spicy foods (such as chilli and curries) should only be eaten in small quantities.

Cook with warming spices such as angelica, black pepper, chilli, cinnamon, garlic, ginger, ginseng, rosemary, wine (your Chinese medicine practitoner will advise on this).

Cold food such as raw fruit and vegetables, ice cream and yoghurt, cucumber, fruit juice, banana.

Anything iced or frozen.

Increasing fruit and vegetables generally is really important.

Pulses Chickpeas, broad beans, lentils, mung beans.

Drinks Green tea, herbal teas such as chamomile, jasmine, mint.

Apples, coconut, lettuce, oats, oyster, pears, watermelon, yoghurt.

Coffee, alcohol, tobacco and other stimulants.

Large quantities of meat, especially red meat.

Deep-fried, roasted and barbecued foods.

All hot spices and spicy food such as chilli, pepper, cinnamon and ginger.

Too much of the allium family (such as garlic, onion, spring onion, leeks).

Earth patterns

Dietary advice

Lifestyle tips

SPLEEN QI AND YANG DEFICIENCY

Eat regular meals – breakfast, lunch and dinner, at regular times.

Avoid overeating, stop before you feel full.

Chew food well and eat slowly.

Focus on your food and the process of eating.

Avoid chilled food and drinks – everything should be room temperature or hotter.

Most foods should be cooked (including fruit). Choose soups, stews, stir-fries and steamed vegetables over raw foods.

Avoid large meals after 6pm.

Focus on simple, easy to digest meals with few ingredients.

Minimise rich food.

Keep your abdomen warm and well covered.

Avoid cold and damp environments where possible.

Take your time to eat in a relaxed environment.

DAMP AND PHLEGM

Avoid foods that have been refined or highly processed, especially fatty and sugary foods.

Eat a higher proportion of vegetables (40–50% of your diet), and relatively less carbohydrates (especially wheat and bread).

Use plenty of digestives in your cooking (such as garlic, mustard, coriander), condiments and relishes (such as pickles, horseradish, mustard, piccalilli).

Avoid overeating, and late night snacks.

Choose good quality oils – in particular olive oil, flax oil, rapeseed oil.

Gentle exercise after eating is helpful.

If you are producing lots of Phlegm on the chest or in your nasal passages, avoid swallowing it.

Beneficial foods	Foods to avoid or reduce

Root vegetables Carrots, celeriac, parsnips, potato, pumpkin, squash, sweet potato.

Grains and pulses Barley, broad beans, chickpeas, maize, millet, oats, peas, rice, soya bean products (tofu, miso, tempeh).

Fruit Cherries, coconut, dates, figs; small amounts of cooked fruits (especially apples, blackberries, cherry, peach).

Animal products (small/moderate amounts only) Beef, chicken, chicken liver (except when pregnant), goose, lamb, mutton, pheasant, pigeon, quail, rabbit.

Seafood Herring, mackerel, mussels, oyster, trout, tuna.

Cabbage and brassicas, celery, chestnuts, oyster mushrooms, walnuts, small amounts of barley malt, molasses, honey.

For Yang Deficiency use warming spices and alliums Basil, cardamom, cayenne, chilli, chive seed, cinnamon, clove, fennel seed, fenugreek, garlic, ginger (especially dried), horseradish, leek, onion, parsley, pepper, nutmeg, rosemary, savory, turmeric.

Large amounts of fruit – choose milder fruits (apples and pears) and warmer fruits (blackberries, cherries, dates, lychee, peach) over tropical fruits (oranges, pineapples, kiwi, melon).

Raw vegetables (including juices).

Foods that are Cold in nature such as ice cream, yoghurt, banana, cucumber, beer.

Anything straight from the fridge or freezer, including iced drinks.

Sugary foods and sweeteners.

Aromatic herbs and alliums Aniseed, basil, caraway, cardamom, chilli (small amounts), clove, coriander, fennel seeds, fenugreek, garlic (small amounts), fresh ginger, horseradish, juniper, mustard, nutmeg, onion, oregano, pepper, rosemary, savory, spring onion, thyme.

Beans and pulses (moderate amounts) Especially aduki beans, broad beans, black beans, chick peas, fava beans, kidney beans, lentils and peas.

Grains Bland grains in moderate amounts such as barley, rye, corn, buckwheat, toasted oats, basmati rice.

Herbal teas Green tea, jasmine tea.

Alfalfa, apples, bamboo shoots, celery, lemons and limes (especially the zest), mushrooms, mustard greens, nori (and other seaweed), olives, pumpkin, radish, shiitake mushroom, turnip, water chestnut, watercress.

Almonds, walnuts and chestnuts are the least Phlegm-forming nuts.

Sugar, sugary food, sweeteners and refined processed foods, especially high carbohydrate food and processed food.

Dairy products Including cheese, butter, yoghurt, ice-cream and milk (goat and sheep products are better).

Fatty foods, especially saturated fats Pork, duck, rich meat.

Poor quality cooking oils.

Peanuts and peanut butter, banana, avocado, wheat.

Yeast products Such as cheese, bread and beer.

Oranges and orange juice.

Nuts, if at all rancid.

Earth patterns continued

Dietary advice	Lifestyle tips

STOMACH YIN DEFICIENCY

Reduce cooking methods that extract moisture such as frying or baking.	Try to eat in a calm and relaxed state and environment whenever possible.

Minimise baked and dry processed foods such as biscuits, crisps and cakes.

Eat regularly: three meals a day, preferably at the same times each day.

Chew food well and eat slowly.

Try to avoid eating your main meal late in the evening, and avoid evening snacking. If possible eat your main meal at lunchtime.

HEAT / FIRE IN THE STOMACH

Increase watery foods (vegetables and fruits).

Eat at regular intervals, and avoid missing meals.

Eat foods that have been cooked in water (soups and casseroles).

If there is physical discomfort, cook food well and favour mashed food and soups until pain subsides.

Drink plenty of fluids, especially water.

Beneficial foods	Foods to avoid or reduce

Fruit All fruit in moderate amounts, especially apples, apricots, banana, kiwi, lychee, peaches, pineapple, plums, citrus in small amounts only (including lemons, oranges, grapefruit, tangerines).

Bamboo shoots, cucumber, spinach, tomatoes, turnip.

If there is Heat in the Stomach, acidic foods may increase indigestion and reflux. In this case it may be necessary to reduce acidic foods (such as citrus, tomato, acidic fruit, coffee, sugar, alcohol, dairy) and increase vegetables.

Alcohol, coffee.

Excessive fatty and deep-fried foods Dairy products, eggs, peanuts, chips, red meat, nuts.

Spicy food and spices such as chilli, pepper, cinnamon and ginger.

Raw garlic or onions.

Lots of vegetables Especially aubergine, avocado, bamboo shoots, bean sprouts, cabbage and other brassicas, celery, cucumber, dandelion, kohlrabi, lettuce, nori and other seaweeds, plantain, potatoes, spinach, chard, water chestnut.

Soups and porridge with well-cooked rice, barley, oats, soya products (tofu, miso, tempeh), goat's milk, goat's yoghurt.

Coffee, alcohol, sugar, tobacco.

Excessive fatty and deep-fried foods Dairy products, eggs, peanuts, chips, red meat (especially beef and lamb), nuts.

Hot and pungent spices Chilli, pepper, ginger, mustard, cinnamon, raw onion, garlic.

Spicy food.

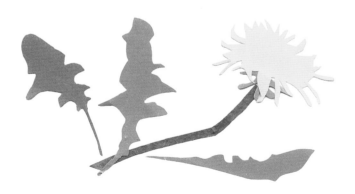

Metal patterns

Dietary advice	Lifestyle tips
LUNG QI DEFICIENCY	
Avoid chilled food and drinks: everything should be room temperature or hotter.	Keep warm and wrapped up – especially your chest, head and neck.
	Regular exercise is essential, especially exercises that expand and open the chest. Breathing exercises are also very useful – consider yoga, tai chi or qi gong.
	Take the appropriate amount of time off to recover from any colds, coughs or infections.
LUNG YIN DEFICIENCY AND DRYNESS	
Avoid over-exercising and drink plenty of fluids when exercising.	Follow the advice given for Lung Qi Deficiency (above) and Stomach Yin Deficiency (page 32).
Preferred cooking methods are steaming, boiling, stewing and stir-frying.	
Minimise dry foods (baked, deep-fried, roasted, barbecued).	
Minimise processed food (biscuits, cakes, crisps and so on).	
PHLEGM IN THE LUNGS	
Avoid overeating and eat simple small regular meals.	A steam inhalation with decongestant essential oils (menthol, eucalyptus) can help.
Use gentle aromatic/spicy flavours in your cooking.	A Neti nasal wash can help to clear the sinuses.
Keep raw foods to a minimum.	
Food and drinks should be served at room temperature or warmer.	
Preferred cooking methods are steaming, boiling, stewing and stir-frying.	

Beneficial foods	Foods to avoid or reduce

Rice (including sweet rice).

Carrots, sweet potato, cabbage and other brassicas, liquorice.

Honey, barley malt and molasses, sparingly.

Small amounts of cooked spicy/pungent foods Onions, garlic, leek, spring onion, horseradish, fresh ginger.

Pork in small amounts.

To strengthen the Qi (immune system) Mushrooms (especially shiitake and ganoderma), honey, royal jelly, lots of fresh fruit and vegetables.

Phlegm forming foods (see Damp and Phlegm, page 31) Dairy, sugar and sweeteners, and so on.

Excess pungent foods (see left) Although small amounts activate the Lung Qi, too much will disperse and weaken it.

Soybean products Tofu, miso, tempeh and soya milk.

Fruit Apple, apricots, banana, fig, grapefruit, peach, pear, strawberry.

Honey, barley malt, rice syrup (in small amounts), almonds, avocado, barley, mushrooms, pine nuts, seaweed, sesame seeds, tahini, hummus, spinach, eggs, mussels, herring, pork.

Dairy products (in small amounts if there is no Phlegm) Yoghurt, cottage cheese, milk, butter; goat and sheep products are easier to digest.

Coffee, alcohol tobacco and other stimulants.

Lamb, chicken, beef.

Too many alliums Such as onion, spring onion, garlic.

Hot spices Such as cinnamon, pepper, ginger, chilli.

Spicy food.

Warming, suitable for Cold conditions Cayenne, chives, fennel seeds, fennel, fenugreek, fresh ginger, garlic, horseradish, leeks, onion, pumpkin, spring onion.

Cooling, suitable for Hot conditions Almonds, grapefruit, lemon, nettles, pear, radish, seaweeds, turnip, water chestnut.

Almonds, walnuts, and chestnuts are the least Phlegm-forming nuts.

See also Damp and Phlegm (page 31).

Sugar, sugary food, sweeteners and refined processed foods.

Dairy products Including cheese, butter, yoghurt and milk (goat and sheep products are better).

Fatty foods Especially saturated fats, pork, duck, rich meat, poor quality oils.

Peanuts and peanut butter, banana, avocado, wheat.

Yeast products Such as cheese, bread and beer.

Oranges and orange juice.

Nuts, if at all rancid.

Water patterns

Dietary advice   **Lifestyle tips**

KIDNEY YANG DEFICIENCY / KIDNEY QI DEFICIENCY

Most foods should be cooked (including fruit). Choose soups, stews, stir-fries and steamed vegetables over raw foods.

Avoid chilled food and drinks – everything should be room temperature or hotter.

Use warming herbs and spices when cooking.

Keep warm; particularly your lower back, feet and abdomen.

Avoid cold and damp environments where possible.

Avoid excessive exercise.

Men should avoid excessive sexual activity.

KIDNEY AND LIVER YIN DEFICIENCY

Reduce cooking methods that extract moisture such as frying or baking.

Minimise baked and dry processed foods such as biscuits, crisps and cakes.

Favour wet food – fruit, salads, steamed and boiled vegetables and leafy greens; soups and stews.

Eat three regular meals a day, preferably at the same time each day.

Chew food well and eat slowly.
Avoid overeating.

Eat a high proportion of fruit and vegetables (40% or more of your diet).

Rest and recovery is the key to whatever you're doing, physically and mentally.

Regular gentle, soft and relaxing exercise is essential.

Avoid late nights, and try to relax in the evening for some time before going to sleep (preferably screen free).

Avoid excessive sweating and keep well hydrated.

Also follow the advice given for Liver Blood Deficiency (page 24).

KIDNEY JING DEFICIENCY / DECLINE IN KIDNEY JING

Avoid over-eating; stop before you are completely full.

Avoid eating late at night; a larger lunch with a smaller evening meal is preferable.

Avoid sudden dietary changes.

Eat regular meals and breakfast.

Men should avoid excessive sexual activity.

Also follow the advice given for Kidney and Liver Yin Deficiency (above).

Beneficial foods	Foods to avoid or reduce

Nuts and seeds Walnuts are especially good. Also chestnuts, pistachios, millet.

Warming herbs/spices Basil, cardamom, cayenne, chilli, chive seed, cinnamon, clove, fennel seed, fenugreek, garlic, dry ginger, horseradish, parsley, pepper, nutmeg, rosemary, savory, turmeric.

Alliums Onions, leeks, spring onions, chives, garlic.

Jasmine tea, grapes, raisins, cherries.

Animal products Anchovy, beef, chicken, kidney, lamb, liver*, lobster, mussels, prawn, shrimp.

With oedema Corn, soya beans, kidney beans, pineapple, carp and mullet.

Uncooked fruit and vegetables (except blackberries and raspberries).

Foods that are Cold in nature such as ice cream, yoghurt, cucumber, fruit juice, banana.

Excessive salt.

Stimulants (including coffee, caffeine, chocolate and recreational drugs).

All fruit Especially apple, apricot, avocado, banana, blackberry, grapefruit, kiwi, lemon, lime, mango, melon, mulberry, peach, pear, pineapple, plum, pomegranate, strawberry, tangerine, watermelon.

Vegetables generally Especially alfalfa, artichoke, asparagus, cucumber, courgette, kohlrabi, nori, plantain, potato, seaweed, squash, sweet potato, tomato, turnip, yam.

All pulses Especially mung beans, butter beans, bean sprouts, kidney beans, miso, tofu, green beans, runner beans.

All nuts and seeds Especially sesame, tahini, pine nut, walnut, coconut milk.

Grains (moderate amounts) Wheat, oats, rice, barley.

Animal products Beef, butter, cheese, eggs, milk, pork, yoghurt.

Seafood Clam, crab, mackerel, mussels, oyster, salmon, sardine, squid.

Alcohol (if you must have a drink, always take it with food).

Coffee, caffeine, stimulants, recreational drugs, tobacco.

Fried foods, saturated fats, excessive animal products (meat and dairy).

Hot spicy food and spices Such as chilli, hot curry, black pepper, raw garlic, raw onions, cinnamon, cloves.

Avoid over-consuming salt.

Animal products (in small, regular amounts) Especially beef, cheese and milk, chicken, duck, eggs, kidney, liver*, mussels, oily fish, pork.

Nuts and seeds Especially almonds, sesame seeds, tahini, sunflower seeds, pumpkin seeds.

Beans and pulses Especially black beans, kidney beans, lentils.

Royal jelly, bee pollen.

* Except during pregnancy, due to high vitamin A

Avoid over-eating animal produce, meat and dairy products.

Coffee, caffeine, alcohol, tobacco.

Refined sugars, processed foods and excessive salt.

Stagnation patterns

Dietary advice	Lifestyle tips

FOOD STAGNATION

Choose a large breakfast, a moderate lunch and a light evening meal whenever possible.

Minimise snacking.

Minimise overeating – stop before you are completely full.

Gentle exercise (such as a short walk) after eating is beneficial, particularly after a large meal.

HEAT STAGNATION

Eat a high proportion of fruit and vegetables (40–50% of your diet) and food with a high water content (soups, stews, salads, steamed and boiled vegetables).

Favour lightly cooked foods (lightly steamed, boiled or stir-fried) over roasted, baked, smoked, deep-fried or barbequed food.

Eat relatively more fish and less red meat.

Reduce cooking methods that extract moisture such as frying or baking.

Minimise baked and dry processed foods such as biscuits, crisps and cakes.

Drink plenty of fluids, especially water.

Fruit and vegetable juices are good in moderate amounts.

Some raw food is beneficial, especially salads.

Avoid overeating.

Follow the advice given for Liver Qi Stagnation (page 26).

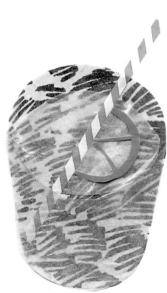

Beneficial foods	Foods to avoid or reduce

Easy to digest foods Soups and stews containing vegetables, well-cooked grains, small amounts of chicken or fish, easy to digest pulses (lentils, miso and tofu, chickpeas, peas).

Digestive herbs Basil, cardamom, cinnamon, cloves, coriander, cumin, ginger, marjoram, mint, nutmeg, oregano, pepper, thyme.

Barley, buckwheat, carrots, coriander, onions, rice, turnips, vinegar.

Young children should avoid wholegrain foods until food Stagnation has resolved.

Moderation in the quantity of rich food such as meat, dairy products, sugars and fats.

Raw foods and food that is difficult to digest (rich fatty foods, excessive amounts of wholemeal and high fibre foods).

Beans and pulses Especially soya products (tofu, miso, soy milk), bean sprouts, mung beans.

All vegetables Especially cucumber, cabbage and brassicas, spinach, celery, potato, lettuce, avocado, bamboo shoots, aubergine, kohlrabi, nori, plantain, chard, water chestnut.

All fruit Especially grapefruit, apples, peaches, plums, apricots, watermelon, kiwi, lemon, tomato (in small quantities).

Grains Rice, barley, oats.

Herbal teas Jasmine, mint or chamomile tea.

Rabbit, clam, crab (in small amounts), goat's milk, goat's yoghurt.

Deep-fried and fatty foods, saturated fats, red meat, beef, pork and lamb.

Roasted or smoked foods.

Shellfish.

Hot spicy food and spices Chilli, cinnamon, horseradish, wasabi, mustard, pepper, raw garlic or onions.

Chocolate, coffee, alcohol (especially spirits), tobacco, other drugs and stimulants.

Excessively salty and sugary food, especially processed food.

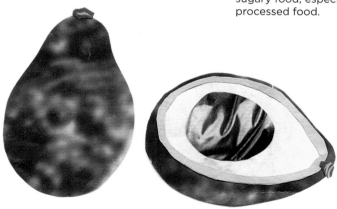

Bowel patterns

Dietary advice   **Lifestyle tips**

CONSTIPATION WITH DRYNESS

Preferred cooking methods are steaming, boiling, soups and stews.

Minimise cooking methods that extract moisture such as frying, roasting or baking, and smoked foods.

Minimise baked and dry processed foods such as biscuits, crisps and cakes.

Eat lots of vegetables and fruit – gradually increase fibre in the diet.

Keep hydrated – drink lots of water, especially after exercise.

PARASITES

Preferred cooking methods are steaming, boiling and stewing.

Wash any raw food/salad well, and use vinegar based dressing.

DIARRHOEA

Preferred cooking methods are steaming boiling, stir-frying.

Avoid all raw foods.

Eat easy to digest foods such as well-cooked grains, soups and stews.

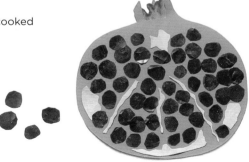

Beneficial foods	Foods to avoid or reduce
Fresh soft vegetables Especially bamboo shoots, carrots, spinach, sweet potato. **Fruit** Especially peaches, pears, bananas, figs, prunes. **Moistening foods** Nuts and seeds generally, especially sesame seeds and tahini, pine nuts, walnuts, almonds, linseeds, honey, wheat bran, rice. **Soups** Made with fresh vegetables, especially the ones above.	Coffee, alcohol. **Fried foods and saturated fats** Especially red meat, beef and lamb. **Hot spices** Chilli, pepper, mustard, cinnamon, raw onion, garlic. Spicy food.
Garlic, celery, pumpkin, pumpkin seeds.	**Mucous-forming foods** Especially sugars and refined foods. Fatty and rich foods and excessive amounts of red meat. **Yeast products** Such as cheese, bread, beer. **Dairy products** Including cheese, butter, yoghurt, milk (goat is better). Oranges and orange juice in large quantities. Wheat.
Black pepper, black tea, buckwheat, chestnut, glutinous rice, lychee, nutmeg, pomegranate fruit and juice, yams.	Excess fruits such as pears, oranges, tangerines, strawberries, plums, kiwis, peaches. Raw fruit and vegetables (cooked fruit and vegetables are fine). Foods that are Cold in nature such as ice cream, yoghurt, banana, and cucumber.

Exterior/Interior patterns

Dietary advice   **Lifestyle tips**

ATTACK OF WIND AND COLD

Eat small simple meals, especially liquid-based foods such as soups and stews.

Drink plenty of water.

Drink savoury tea (see opposite), then have a hot shower or bath and go to bed well covered up. If there is little change, drink more tea when you wake and rest.

Honey, ginger and lemon tea (see opposite) will help alleviate symptoms during the day.

Allow plenty of time to fully recuperate after a cold.

ATTACK OF WIND AND HEAT

Eat small simple meals, especially liquid-based foods such as soups and stews.

Fruit juice and smoothies are useful.

Drink tea (see opposite) then have a hot shower or bath and go to bed well covered up. If there is little change, drink more tea when you wake and then rest.

FULL HEAT/HEAT IN THE QI LEVEL

Eat small simple meals, especially liquid-based foods such as soups and stews.

Fruit juice and smoothies are useful.

Avoid fried, roasted, smoked or barbecued foods.

WITH DAMPNESS/SPLEEN QI DEFICIENCY

WITH PHLEGM HEAT/DAMP HEAT

Beneficial foods	Foods to avoid or reduce

Broccoli, cabbage, carrots, cooked fruit, coriander, garlic, lemon juice, parsnips, spring onions.

Savoury tea Simmer the following for 5 minutes in 300ml water: 20g each fresh ginger root, garlic, spring onion and 10g cayenne pepper. Strain the liquid off. Mix with 2 tsps brown sugar and drink.

Honey, ginger and lemon tea Add 1 lemon (juice and zest), 25–50mm grated fresh ginger and 1 tbsp honey to 600ml boiling water. Strain and drink.

Herbs (use in a soup or stew) Black pepper, chilli, cinnamon twig, garlic, fresh ginger, horseradish.

Rich and greasy food
Dairy, meat and deep-fried foods.

Fruit Especially lemon juice, grapefruit.

Vegetables Broccoli, cabbage, carrots, parsnips.

Herbal tea Simmer the following for 3 minutes in 300ml water: 10g each of chamomile, peppermint and chrysanthemum. Strain the liquid off and drink.

Alternatively drink green, mint or chamomile tea.

Rich and greasy food
Dairy, meat and deep-fried foods.

Bananas, Chinese cabbage, mung beans, pears, plums, rice, turnips, water chestnuts, watermelon.

Pungent foods Including all onions, garlic, chillies and ginger.

Alcohol, coffee.

Oily, greasy and fried foods Especially beef and lamb.

Barley water Simmer 100g of barley in 600ml water for 30 minutes. Pour off the liquid. Drink it with your meal, and eat the barley.

Avoid mucous-forming foods (see Damp and Phlegm, page 31).

Apple, cabbage, carrot, cauliflower, mushroom, papaya, pear, pumpkin, radish, strawberry, watercress.

Rich and greasy food Dairy, meat and deep-fried foods.

Coffee, alcohol.

Onions, garlic.

Hot spices Such as cinnamon, pepper, dry ginger, chilli.

Other dietary considerations

Cholesterol

Cholesterol is incredibly important to us; it is essential for brain and general cell function, hormone production and balance. Levels may become raised in some people for no apparent reason (primary, or inherited) or because of diet and lifestyle (secondary, or acquired).

Chinese medicine regards high cholesterol as thickening of Blood and body fluids, and the development of Phlegm. To regulate this imbalance, circulation should be increased (through regular exercise), and Phlegm should be reduced (through specific dietary changes – see Liver Qi Stagnation, page 26, Liver Fire, page 26 and Damp and Phlegm, page 30).

Other long-term dietary changes to help reduce cholesterol include:

1 Replacing foods that are high in saturated fats (fatty meats, cakes, biscuits, cheese and butter) with foods that are high in unsaturated fats such as oily fish (mackerel and salmon), nuts (almonds and walnuts), seeds (sunflower and pumpkin) and vegetable oils (olive, walnut and rapeseed).

2 Slowly and gradually increasing soluble fibre by eating more fruit and vegetables, and increasing foods like oats, barley, beans, peas, lentils and chickpeas.

3 Adding beneficial foods and drinks to our diet including green tea, soya products, apples, garlic and hawthorn.

Important note We advise you to have your cholesterol levels monitored by your GP, as well as seeking advice from an acupuncturist or Chinese herbal medicine practitioner (see Finding a Chinese medicine practitioner near you, page 48).

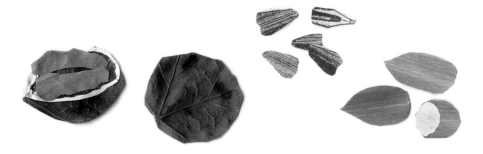

Minerals [6, 7, 8]

Calcium Enrich your intake by eating dairy products; nuts; seeds; pulses and soya bean products; leafy greens; dried fruits (raisins, prunes, figs, apricots); bony fish (sardines, pilchards); fortified products (bread, breakfast cereal, soya and rice milk); parsley, swede, and mushrooms. Too much salt (such as processed foods, crisps), protein (excessive meat and dairy produce) and caffeine (tea, coffee, fizzy drinks) can increase the amount of calcium your body loses. Regular weight-bearing exercise and stopping smoking aids absorption, as does **Vitamin D**, so 'sensible' sunshine and foods like oily fish (salmon, sardines, and mackerel); eggs; butter and fortified products (such as spreads and breakfast cereal) are also important.

Magnesium Eat plenty of green leafy vegetables (including all green and root vegetables, especially spinach and avocados); nuts and seeds (especially pumpkin seeds, cashew nuts); fish (especially mackerel and shellfish); beans and lentils; wholemeal grains; chocolate, beer; bananas and figs.

Potassium Good sources include virtually all unprocessed plant and animal foods; dark leafy greens; fruits (bananas, apricots); nuts and seeds; wheat bran; fish (salmon, tuna) and mushrooms.

Iron Good sources include all kinds of meat including poultry, fish and especially liver (avoid liver during pregnancy due to high vitamin A levels); beans and pulses (especially lentils, chickpeas, kidney beans, soya bean products, tofu); leafy greens (all, especially cabbage and spinach); nuts and seeds (especially sunflower seeds, pumpkin seeds, sesame seeds, almonds, cashews); dried fruit (especially apricots, prunes, figs, dates, raisins); wholemeal grains, brown rice, millet, wheat germ; molasses and parsley.

Iron levels are reduced by long or hot cooking methods. The amount of iron you can absorb is reduced by drinking tea, coffee, hot chocolate or red wine with a meal and by including lots of grains, dairy products, soya products, oregano or chocolate.

Iron absorption is increased by including vitamin C (fresh vegetables or fruit) in your meal, cooking in a heavy iron pan, and by fermenting foods.

Zinc Good sources include nuts and seeds (especially almonds, pumpkin seeds, sesame seeds and cashews); wholemeal grains; beans and pulses (especially lentils); dark chocolate; mushrooms; meat (beef, lamb, chicken); fish and shellfish; dairy products; eggs; root vegetables and leafy greens.

Substitute foods

Milk Try soya milk, rice milk, almond milk, coconut milk or goat's milk.

Cheese Try tofu, tempeh, nut cheese, soya cheese, goat's cheese or sheep's cheese.

Yoghurt Try soya, rice or goat's milk yoghurt.

Butter Use olive, rapeseed or coconut oil.

Wheat Oats and oat products; corn and corn products (corn thins, popcorn); rye and rye bread; buckwheat; rice and rice products (rice cakes). Spelt is easier to digest than other wheat varieties. Try vegetable or rice pasta and flour. Many gluten-free products are now available – these are easier to digest.

Coffee and tea Try herbal teas like mint, rosehip and hibiscus, chamomile, fennel, liquorice, jasmine, green tea or rooibos. Visit your local shops and healthfood shops where you'll find many healthier alternatives.

Meat Use pulses like chickpeas, lentils or kidney beans in place of mince or in curries, soups and stews. Try quorn, tofu, tempeh and pulses instead of beef or chicken. Make nut roasts or pies in place of roasted joints. If using beans and pulses as a protein, combine with a carbohydrate food to ensure a 'complete protein'.

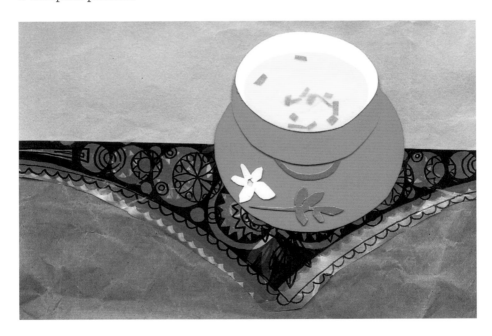

Boosting your Qi (immune system)

Here is a list of the best foods to boost your Qi (immune system) from a variety of sources – they may contain high levels of vitamin C, carotenoids, bioflavonoids or other antioxidant ingredients.

Vegetables Avocado, beetroot, broccoli, cabbage, carrot, cauliflower, chives, garlic, kale, leafy greens, leek, lettuce, onion, parsnip, peas, pepper, potato, pumpkin, shallots, shiitake mushroom, spinach, squash, sweet potato, sweetcorn, tomato, watercress.

Fruit Apples, apricot, banana, blackberry, blackcurrants, blueberry, cherry, cranberry, date, gouji berries, grape, grapefruit, guava, kiwi, lemon, longan, mango, melon, nectarine, orange, papaya, pear, pineapple, strawberry, watermelon.

Nuts and seeds Almond, bean sprouts (all kinds), cashew, chia seeds, linseed, pine nuts, pistachio, pumpkin seeds, sesame seeds, sunflower seeds, tahini, walnut.

Grains and pulses Amaranth, quinoa, barley, buckwheat, butterbeans, chickpeas, lentils, millet, oats, popcorn, rice, soya (including tofu, miso, tempeh and tamari), wheatgerm.

Drinks and sweet things Green tea, honey, manuka honey, molasses, dark chocolate (at least 80% cacao).

Herbs and spices Cinnamon, cloves, coriander, garlic, fresh ginger, mint, parsley, rosemary, thyme, turmeric.

Acid-forming and alkaline-forming foods

Acid-forming foods Red meat, processed foods (cereals, cakes, biscuits, and other foods with high sugar and salt content or refined carbohydrates), sugary drinks (fizzy drinks, cola), coffee, tea, chocolate, alcohol, acidic fruits (citrus, tomatoes).

Alkaline-forming foods Dates, figs, apricots, apple, pear, mango, papaya, avocado, lemon, lime, watercress, fennel, asparagus, celery, cauliflower, onion, garlic, fresh ginger and beetroot, kelp, spinach, rocket, parsley, coriander, sunflower, pumpkin and sesame seeds (and their oils), almonds, walnuts, pecans, quinoa, millet, buckwheat, oats, brown rice, almond milk, brown rice, coconut water.

Notes

1 Le QT, Elliott WJ, 'Hypotensive and hypocholesterolemic effects of celery oil may be due to BuPh', *Clin Res*, 1991;39:173A.

2 Tse, G, Eslick, GD, 'Cruciferous vegetables and risk of colorectal neoplasms: a systematic review and meta-analysis', *Nutrition and Cancer* 66 (1): 128–139, 2014 doi:10.1080/01635581.2014.852686. PMID 24341734

3 Borchers, AT, Krishnamurthy, A, Keen, CL, Meyers, FJ, Gershwin, ME, 'The immunobiology of mushrooms', *Experimental Biology and Medicine* 233 (3): 259–76, 2008 doi:10.3181/0708-MR-227. PMID 18296732

4 cancerresearchuk.org/about-cancer/cancers-in-general/cancer-questions/mushrooms-in-cancer-treatment

5 nhs.uk/conditions/lactose-intolerance

6 *Vitamin and Mineral Requirements in Human Nutrition*, World Health Organization, 2004, ISBN 92 4 154612 3

7 nhs.uk/conditions/vitamins-minerals/pages/vitamins-minerals.aspx

8 vegsoc.org/facts/vitaminsminerals

Finding a Chinese medicine practitioner near you

British Acupuncture Council
63 Jeddo Road, London W12 9HQ
020 8735 0400   acupuncture.org.uk

Register of Chinese Herbal Medicine
Office 6, 27 Castle Meadow,
Norwich, NR1 3DS
01603 623994   rchm.co.uk

College of Integrated Chinese Medicine
19 Castle Street, Reading, RG1 7SB
0118 950 8880   cicm.org.uk

Further reading

For interested patients

Helping Ourselves: A Guide to Traditional Chinese Food Energetics, Daverick Leggett, Meridian Press, ISBN 978-0-9524640-0-6

Recipes for Self-Healing, Daverick Leggett, Meridian Press, ISBN 978-0-9524640-2-0

Be Your Own Nutritionist, George Cooper, Short Books, ISBN 978-1-78072-156-9

For interested practitioners

Healing with Whole Foods, Paul Pitchford, North Atlantic Books, ISBN 1-55643-220-8

Clinical Handbook of Internal Medicine Volume 2 – Spleen and Stomach, Will Maclean and Jane Lyttleton, University of Western Sydney, ISBN 978-095797200-1

Chinese Nutrition Therapy: Dietetics in Traditional Chinese Medicine, Joerg Kastner, Thieme Paperback, ISBN 978-3131309624

Chinese Dietary Therapy, Liu Jilin and Gordon Peck, Churchill Livingstone, ISBN 0-443-04967-X

Prince Wen Hui's Cook, Bob Flaws and Honora Wolfe, Paradigm Publications, ISBN 0-912111-05-4